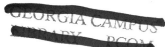

2008–2009
Medical Student's Guide to Successful Residency Matching

D0877745

2008–2009

Medical Student's Guide to Successful Residency Matching

Lee T. Miller, MD

Cedars-Sinai Medical Center
Professor of Pediatrics
Vice Chair of Education
Department of Pediatrics
David Geffen School of Medicine at UCLA
Los Angeles, California

Leigh B. Grossman, MD

Professor of Pediatrics
Chief, Division of Infectious Disease
Department of Pediatrics
University of Virginia School of Medicine
Charlottesville, Virginia

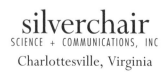

silverchair
SCIENCE + COMMUNICATIONS, INC
Charlottesville, Virginia

To order additional copies of this book, please visit your health science bookstore or www.rittenhouse.com.

Publisher: Silverchair Science + Communications, Inc.
Printer: RR Donnelley, Harrisonburg, VA

Printed in the United States of America.

9 8 7 6 5 4 3 2 1

ISBN-10: 0-9787436-2-8
ISBN-13: 978-0-9787436-2-8

Contents

Preface

There are over 25,000 individuals applying for residency training in the United States, and such individuals are faced with the enormous task of selecting from a wide variety of graduate medical education training programs. It is our goal to guide the applicant through the year-long matching process with a step-by-step guide to successful residency matching from start to finish. The scope of this book encompasses specialty selection, curriculum planning for the third and fourth years of medical school, program selection for residency application, strategies for interviewing and ranking, tips for the international medical graduate, and an overview of the different matching programs, with particular emphasis on the National Resident Matching Program.

We would like to thank the thousands of students from across the country over the last 20 years whose enthusiastic comments, suggestions, and questions have helped us strengthen this project. This book was written with the spirit and hope that we can help tomorrow's house officers match successfully with the residency programs of their choosing.

Lee T. Miller, MD
Leigh B. Grossman, MD

Acknowledgments

We would again like to express our sincere appreciation to the students who continue to ask the questions and seek the best possible residency training. Their passion, enthusiasm, and dedication remain the inspiration and motivation for this guide. In particular, we would like to thank Jeff Donowitz, a second year student whose insights have been invaluable.

We would like to express our tremendous gratitude once again to Mona M. Signer, the Executive Director of the National Resident Matching Program, and to Stephen Seeling, the Vice President for Operations of the Educational Commission for Foreign Medical Graduates, for their review and contributions to this manuscript.

We also wish to thank Arlene Estrada, whose dedication, organization, editorial and administrative expertise, patience, and sense of humor continue to make this a far better book.

Choosing Your Medical Specialty

Choosing which medical specialty to pursue is a career decision that carries with it a lifetime commitment to care for specific patients with specific diseases. Most students consider this the most important and most difficult decision they make during their medical school years. Some specialists will only deliver babies, only see children, only psychoanalyze, only read radiographs, only examine skin, or only examine eyes. These different specialties also carry with them a certain professional identity that may influence such things as lifestyle and friends, particularly in this time of rapid change in our health care world. Be certain that you take the time to find advisors at all levels of their careers who can describe the profession today, and, it is hoped, project for you where the profession may be tomorrow.

ADVISORS FOR SPECIALTY DECISION-MAKING

As a medical student, you may have family members who can provide you with historical and current information on different medical specialties. This advice can be extremely useful because these individuals may be able to incorporate knowledge of your background and personality into the discussion. However, this advice can also be extremely pressured and biased. When a parent or family member has strong feelings about your choice of specialty, the counsel may be a detriment to your freedom of decision-making. It is important that you make your own decision, realizing that any parental or familial disappointment now will later disappear when a happier son or daughter has fulfilled his or her own goals.

Alumni of your school or its residency programs who teach or practice in the area may be extremely useful advisors. They may better understand your educational background and can speak freely of their own decisions and whether their goals have been realized.

Present house officers and chief residents in particular specialties are usually wonderful advisors because they can very accurately reflect on their recent decision-making. They can also comment on the pros and cons of the specific and current residency training requirements and potential employment opportunities upon completion of training.

The Dean of Students may be a good advisor on specialty choice, but is unlikely to be able to offer much specific information on residency programs in a particular discipline unless he or she is specifically trained in that field.

A faculty advisor can be extremely helpful, but again, becomes more useful when you are asking about this advisor's own field of expertise. It is more important to utilize the experience of the faculty advisor after you have chosen a specialty and are seeking more information on that career, residency training, and specific training programs within that particular specialty (see Chapter 4).

REALITIES OF YOUR SPECIALTY CHOICE

It is extremely important that you fully understand the training requirements, the career possibilities, and the lifestyle realities of the specialty you are considering.

Requirements

The minimum training requirements to meet Board eligibility in most specialties are outlined in Table 1.1. Individual program requirements may differ from these minimum Board requirements, including additional years of clinical work and/or research. Specialty training programs in family practice, pediatrics, and internal medicine appear to have a shorter training period (usually 3 years) when compared with the surgical subspecialties. However, if you decide to further subspecialize, then during your residency years in pediatrics, internal medicine, or family practice you will apply for additional subspecialty fellowship training (e.g., in pediatric allergy, cardiology, critical care, endocrinology, gastroenterology, hematology/oncology, infectious disease, neonatology, nephrology, or pulmonology). Training will then be 6 years (3 years of pediatric residency training plus 3 years of pediatric subspeciality fellowship training). This training period, then, is not very different from the length of time required to complete general surgery training. The *Graduate Medical Education Directory* lists requirements for specialty and subspecialty training in all fields, and we encourage you to familiarize yourself with the wide variety of residency and potential subspecialty training opportunities available to you.

Career Opportunities

Consideration of the availability of positions upon completion of training is a necessary part of this decision. It is important to determine whether opportunities will be available to practice your academic or private specialty, or whether a given field is already too competitive and saturated.

Lifestyle

An accurate assessment of what effect your career choice will have on your personal lifestyle is also imperative. Weekly hours, nighttime and weekend duties, geographic location, financial compensation, malpractice insurance costs, and many other lifestyle factors will be greatly influenced by this career decision. It is important to envision as much of this as possible and truthfully acknowledge your own personal needs and priorities as you make this decision.

Once you have sorted through the above, keep in mind that the future of many specialties is impossible to predict. Many of the medical fields have markedly changed in the last 20 to 30 years and may continue to do so. Radiology, for example, is a field that has enjoyed tremendous growth. As you know, the radiologist is no longer limited to just the black and white roentgenogram. This discipline now includes subspecialties in angiography, ultrasonography, magnetic resonance imaging, and nuclear scanning. The primary care specialties have also undergone impressive growth. Although changes in specialties are difficult to predict, personal preferences on what kind of people you wish to serve and in what setting you wish to practice will probably not change radically with time. Therefore, the rotations in which you are most comfortable during your third and fourth years probably reflect an environment that you will enjoy for a long time. This "gut feeling," or comfort level, should carry significant weight in your decision-making.

SPECIALTY COMPETITION

It is important to determine your competitiveness or "how good you look" compared with the rest of your class and other students competing for similar positions from all over the country. If you are a superb student at a small, relatively lesser known school, if you can obtain excellent letters of reference, and if you have strong interview skills showing your directedness and dedication, then you should apply to your top choices regardless of how competitive these medical centers or specialties may be. If you are in the middle of your class even at a renowned institution, you will need strong letters of recommendation and excellent interviews to obtain your top choices. It is important, however, that you list your strengths and weaknesses and understand your class rank and competitiveness so that you neither underestimate nor overestimate your abilities.

It is also important that you assess the competitiveness of the programs to which you are applying. Some specialties have many unfilled places each year, and, in these fields, you should not be afraid to aim high for a strong residency position. We recommend that you apply both to excellent programs where your chances of securing a position are not high but still possible, and also to other places on your list that are good, solid, but less competitive programs, where you have a higher likelihood of successful matching. The matching system, as it was established, possibly allows you to do better than you would through a routine acceptance situation, particularly in the less competitive specialties. In highly competitive programs, it is much more important to assess your class standing very accurately and have the chairman or a faculty member with expertise in this specialty honestly assess your likelihood of success in securing a residency position in this field. Particularly in specialties with very small numbers of positions (e.g., dermatology, orthopedics, and neurosurgery), it is extremely important to find out if you are competitive for one of these positions.

It is suggested that you be well along in this career decision-making process by the early fall of your senior year.

OTHER TIPS FOR SPECIALTY SELECTION

For those of you who, during the summer before your final year, find yourselves still not knowing which career direction you'd like to pursue, we'd like to urge you to relax. It may become increasingly more difficult for you to maintain your composure while more and more friends share with you their excitement over their own career decisions. Please remember that this is not a race, and your time will come soon enough. There are, however, several things we can suggest that might help you to reach a decision sooner rather than later.

Most important, we urge you to take advantage of the flexibility of your senior year to re-explore specialty areas that you may be considering. This is your chance to "retest the waters" before making your final decisions. You may have a very different impression when you revisit a service as a senior student on an elective or subinternship. You will likely no longer share the worries of the third-year students on your service (e.g., presentations on rounds, preparations for final exams) and can focus your energies instead on trying to feel what it would be like to dedicate your career to that particular specialty.

If you're considering more than one specialty during the summer before your final year, you might also want to review information from more than one type of residency training program. Often, when learning in greater detail about the specifics of each training program, students may find themselves pulled in one direction rather than another, and they may also find themselves more excited about a particular type of training program. Once you do make your specialty choice, you'll be ready to complete the application materials in a timely fashion, having already solicited materials from programs earlier in your decision-making process.

While some students look for as many reasons as possible to put off writing their personal statement, we might even suggest that you consider more than one— that is, a different personal statement for each specialty area that you're considering. Many students have found this to be an extremely revealing exercise when they have difficulty articulating on paper all of the reasons why they might want to pursue specialty "A" versus the ease with which they can explain on paper all of the reasons for pursuing specialty "B."

Regardless of how and when you choose which specialty you'd like to pursue, we can't emphasize enough how important it is that you and you alone make this decision. You're the one who will have to roll out of bed at 5:30 or 6:00 in the morning to prepare for work rounds, not your many friends or family members who are urging you to pursue various directions. Once again, the bottom line here is that only you can make this decision from your heart.

TABLE 1.1
*Training Requirements by Specialty**

Specialty	Preliminary Track Training (years)	Minimum Required Length of Specialty Residency Training for Board Eligibility (years)	Minimum Total Number of Years of Training to Meet Board Eligibility Requirements	Application Deadline
Anesthesiology	1 (Optional for some Anesthesiology programs)	3	4	Apply to Anesthesiology programs 2 years before beginning your training in Anesthesiology
Colon and Rectal Surgery	5 (General Surgery)	1	6	Apply to Colon and Rectal Surgery programs 1–2 years before beginning your training in Colon and Rectal Surgery
Dermatology	1	3	4	Apply to Dermatology programs 2 years before beginning your training in Dermatology
Emergency Medicine (EM)	1 (Optional for some EM programs)	3	3	Apply to EM programs 2 years in advance if applying for preliminary training first; otherwise, apply 1 year in advance if EM program incorporates an internship

Family Practice	0	3	3	Apply to Family Practice programs 1 year before beginning your training in Family Practice
Internal Medicine	0	3	3	Apply to Internal Medicine programs 1 year before beginning your training in Internal Medicine
Neurology[1]	1 (>8 months Internal Medicine)	3	4	Apply to Neurology programs 2 years before beginning your training in Adult Neurology
Child Neurology	1–2 (Pediatrics and/or Research year)	3	5	Apply via the San Francisco Matching Program to Child Neurology programs 2 years before beginning your training in Child Neurology
Neurologic Surgery	1	5	6	Apply to Neurosurgery programs 2 years before beginning your training in Neurosurgery

(continued)

TABLE 1.1—*continued*

Specialty	Preliminary Track Training (years)	Minimum Required Length of Specialty Residency Training for Board Eligibility (years)	Minimum Total Number of Years of Training to Meet Board Eligibility Requirements	Application Deadline
Nuclear Medicine	2	2	4	Apply for Nuclear Medicine during your preliminary track clinical training 1–2 years before beginning training in Nuclear Medicine
Obstetrics-Gynecology (OB-GYN)	1 (Optional)	3 or 4	4	Apply to OB-GYN programs 1 year in advance if applying to a 4-year OB-GYN program
Ophthalmology	1	3	4	Apply via the San Francisco Matching Program to Ophthalmology programs 2 years before beginning your training in Ophthalmology
Orthopedic Surgery	1 (Optional for some Orthopedic Surgery programs)	4	5	Apply to Orthopedic Surgery programs 2 years before beginning your training in Orthopedic Surgery

Specialty				Comments
Otolaryngology	1–2	4	5	Apply to Otolaryngology programs 2 years before beginning your training in Otolaryngology (or 3 years for programs requiring 2 years of General Surgery training)
Pathology (Combined Anatomical and Clinical)	0	5	5	Apply to Pathology programs 1 year before beginning your training in Pathology
Pediatrics	0	3	3	Apply to Pediatrics programs in the fall 1 year before beginning your training in Pediatrics
Physical Medicine and Rehabilitation (PM and R)	1 (Optional for some Physical Medicine and Rehabilitation programs)	3–4	4	Apply to PM and R programs 1 year in advance if going into a program that incorporates preliminary training
Plastic Surgery[2]	3 (General Surgery)	2	5	Apply to Plastic Surgery programs 2 years before beginning your Plastic Surgery training (with application routes through both the NRMP and San Francisco Matching Program)

(continued)

TABLE 1.1—*continued*

Specialty	Preliminary Track Training (years)	Minimum Required Length of Specialty Residency Training for Board Eligibility (years)	Minimum Total Number of Years of Training to Meet Board Eligibility Requirements	Application Deadline
Preventive Medicine	1	1	2 (Residency must be followed by a year of field work to meet Board eligibility requirements)	Apply directly to Preventive Medicine programs 1 year before beginning your preliminary year training
Psychiatry	1	3	4	Apply to Psychiatry programs 1 year in advance if program includes preliminary training; otherwise, 2 years before beginning your training in Psychiatry
Radiology	1 (Optional for some Radiology programs)	4	5	Apply to Radiology programs 2 years before beginning your training in Radiology
Surgery (General)	0	5	5	Apply to General Surgery programs 1 year before beginning your training in Surgery

Thoracic Surgery	2–3	5	7	Apply to Thoracic Surgery programs 2 years before beginning your training in Thoracic Surgery
Urology	2	3	5	Apply via the American Urologic Association to Urology programs 1–2 years before beginning your training in Urology
Vascular Surgery	1–2	5	6	Apply to Vascular Surgery programs 1 year before beginning your Integrated Vascular Surgery Residency or 2 or 4 years into your General Surgery Residency.

[1] Adult Neurology has a "Two-Tier Match" designed to serve those students who are ready to choose Neurology in January of their senior year as well as those who wish to postpone their decision until January of their PGY-1 year.

[2] Some plastic surgery positions are offered at the PGY-1 level through the NRMP Match. These positions are "integrated" and provide 3 years of General Surgery training and 2 years of Plastic Surgery training. Most positions in Plastic Surgery are filled in a separate match in May of the PGY-2 year or later (14 months before the start of Plastic Surgery training).

Note: Individual program requirements may differ from these minimum board requirements, including additional years of clinical work and/or research. Please also check with individual Specialty Boards for the most updated information on training requirements.

SUGGESTED READINGS

American Medical Association. *Graduate Medical Education Directory (GMED)*, Chicago, current edition (annual publication referred to as the "Green Book," available for online purchase at *http://www.ama-assn.org/ama/pub/category/3991.html*).

Careers in Medicine (CiM), hosted by the Association of American Medical Colleges. Available at: *http://www.aamc.org/students/cim/start.htm*.

Choosing a Specialty, hosted by the American Medical Association. Available at: *http://www.ama-assn.org/ama/pub/category/7247.html*.

Fellowship and Residency Electronic Interactive Database (FREIDA Online) hosted by the American Medical Association. Available at: *http://www.ama-assn.org/ama/pub/category/2997.html*.

Freeman BS. *The Ultimate Guide to Choosing a Medical Specialty*. New York: Lange Medical Books, 2004.

Iserson KV. *Iserson's Getting into a Residency: A Guide for Medical Students*. 7th ed., Galen Press, Tucson, AZ, 2006.

Medical Careers: Career Advising and Planning Program Developed Jointly by the AAMC and the AMA, 1999. Available at: *http://www.aamc.org/students/cim/specialties.htm*.

Medical Specialty Aptitude Test, hosted by Dr. Peter Filsinger, et al. 2006. Available at: *http://www.med-ed.virginia.edu/specialities*.

Stein J. *Impact on Personal Life Key to Choosing a Medical Specialty in the '80's*. Internal Medicine World Report, 1988:3;7.

Strolling Through the Match, hosted by the American Academy of Family Physicians 2006–2007. Available at: *http://aafp.org/online/en/home/publications/otherpubs/strolling.html*.

Taylor AD. *How to Choose a Medical Specialty*. 4th ed. W.B. Saunders, Co., Philadelphia, 2003.

Planning Your Clinical Years

THE THIRD YEAR OF MEDICAL SCHOOL— CLERKSHIP SCHEDULING

Many second-year medical students will be given the opportunity to bid on the sequence of their third-year clinical clerkships. We'd like to stress that the order of your rotations will ultimately have little impact upon your overall performance, and that there are advantages and disadvantages to starting on more or less rigorous services. However, if you are approaching your third year of medical school with a particular favorite specialty in mind, it may be in your best interest to avoid doing this specialty rotation at the very start of your third year. Remember that your first weeks to months on the wards will be spent "learning the ropes" of being a clinical clerk, including presentations, histories and physicals, venipuncture and other procedures, and learning your way around the hospital(s). Although by no means a hard-and-fast rule, you are much more likely to "shine" a bit later in your third year when you are more polished and comfortable with your new clinical responsibilities. Similarly, some students advocate that you should also avoid scheduling your favorite clerkships at the very end of the third year when you are more likely to be exhausted from the rigors of the preceding 9 to 12 months. However, we would like to emphasize again that regardless of the sequence of your clinical clerkships, you will have multiple opportunities to demonstrate your abilities and to perform admirably.

THE THIRD YEAR OF MEDICAL SCHOOL— CLERKSHIP LOCATIONS

Most medical schools will offer their students opportunities to rotate through services at either a home institution (usually a university hospital) or multiple affiliated centers, which may vary from tertiary care centers, to community hospitals, to outlying clinics, to Veterans Administration hospitals, to county or public facilities, and to Health Maintenance Organization settings. Regardless of your clerkship assignments, the most important thing is to strive for excellence on your clinical rotations. You will undoubtedly face several non-ideal and otherwise difficult situations along the way. For example, a poor attending physician, a weak resident, or a county health care facility with poorly funded ancillary services may present obstacles. Despite this, you will do yourself a disservice by allowing your environment to adversely affect your attitude, and thus, to result in less than your best performance. Furthermore, if you feel slighted that you have missed an opportunity to work with the faculty at your home institution in your specialty of interest, you will have ample occasions to demonstrate your abilities on elective opportunities throughout your senior year.

THE FOURTH YEAR OF MEDICAL SCHOOL— REQUIRED ROTATIONS, ELECTIVE TIME, EXTRAMURAL ELECTIVES, AND INTERVIEW SCHEDULING

Be sure to check with your Dean's Office for a list of required rotations for your fourth year of medical school. At the same time, you may inquire as to the maximum number of rotations that may be taken away from your home institution. In most instances, the majority of your last year of medical school may be spent on clinical or research electives. Your fourth year should not be perceived as unimportant just because it affords flexibility and the opportunity to pursue elective training. Rather, this year should be viewed as a valuable opportunity to solidify your clinical skills and fund of knowledge and to broaden your foundation in medicine. Furthermore, for those students who start their fourth year leaning toward a particular specialty choice, your early electives are a great opportunity to reaffirm this decision. For those students wrestling between two or more specialties, these early electives will allow you to retest the waters with a very different perspective as a senior student. For some specialties, it may be more important than others that you pursue research opportunities to demonstrate your enthusiasm. Be sure to discuss your plans and elective choices well in advance with your faculty advisor, and perhaps with other more senior students who are preparing for graduation.

In planning your senior year, you should plan to have at least 2 to 4 weeks without any scheduled rotations for interviewing. In most cases the interview season will begin after November 1 when your Medical Student Performance Evaluation (MSPE, formerly known as the "Dean's Letter of Recommendation") is mailed out, and extends through late January. The time required to complete your interviews will vary, of course, depending upon the geographic spread of the programs to which you are applying. In addition to the 2 to 4 weeks that you dedicate to interviews in your fourth year schedule, most elective supervisors and attending physicians will understand if you request occasional additional days off for interviewing at other times during the late fall or winter months, provided these requests are not excessive. We also recommend a light schedule filled with less rigorous electives at the end of your fourth year (i.e., after Match Day). You will enjoy having more leisure time to relax and unwind before your internship, and will appreciate a lighter schedule as you begin making plans for finding a new home, packing, and moving.

An "acting internship" or "subinternship" in your specialty of choice will significantly add to your credentials and strengthen your recommendation if you perform admirably. Such rotations are not only excellent teaching opportunities, but also confidence builders as you approach the end of medical school and the beginning of your internship. At the same time, it is crucial to maintain a sense of balance throughout your fourth year by rotating through multiple disciplines. Please do not try to mimic your internship as a senior student by taking more than three or four electives in your specialty of choice. Rather, we recommend that you take advantage of this valuable elective time in multiple disciplines to broaden your foundation and breadth of experience in clinical medicine. For example, a critical care rotation will help all students improve their organizational skills and expertise with procedures. Similarly, a rotation on a radiology service, in an emergency room, or on an anesthesiology service should provide valuable teaching for all students pursuing any kind of clinical training.

"Extramural electives" or "audition electives" (i.e., electives at institutions other than your medical school or its closely affiliated centers) can either help or hinder your application for residency at that center. A less-than-strong performance at another institution will markedly lessen your chances for matching at that institution. We do not recommend extramural rotations solely for the purpose of impressing a residency selection committee unless your faculty advisor believes that it is in your best interest for a particularly competitive specialty or program. If you are a superb student, for the majority of specialties at least, you will likely be able to match in one of your top choice programs without rotating there on an extramural elective. On the other hand, rotations at other institutions provide tremendous opportunities to:

- Learn more about a particular type of institution (e.g., rotating through a children's hospital versus a general university hospital versus a community hospital).
- Learn more about a particular geographic area in which you're considering relocating for your internship.
- Learn more about a particular discipline on a stronger teaching service than your home institution can offer (e.g., rotating on a strong hematology-oncology service with a fine reputation for teaching).

We also recommend that you take advantage of the many unique opportunities afforded to senior medical students (e.g., rotations in Alaska, rotations with the U.S. Public Health service in rural settings, clinical experiences in developing nations, etc.), provided your overall curriculum is well balanced and meets all requirements for graduation. Many medical schools will assign a faculty advisor to counsel students on international elective opportunities and who might also be able to direct students toward resources for funding.

In summary, your fourth year of medical school offers tremendous opportunities to broaden your knowledge base in multiple disciplines, while allowing you to sort out and solidify career choices and explore internship opportunities. Elective planning should be carefully reviewed and discussed with your faculty advisor as you embark on this exciting and enriching last year of your undergraduate medical education.

TIMETABLE FOR THE THIRD AND FOURTH YEAR

It is critical that you understand the application timetable as you plan your schedule for your fourth year of medical school. For example, for most specialties you will need to have a dedicated block of time between November and January for interviews, and as mentioned above, most students block out 2 to 4 weeks of vacation between November and January for this purpose. However, for a small subset of specialties, the entire application, interview, and ranking processes occur early (sometimes referred to as "early match specialties"), and you need to plan accordingly so that you are able to schedule all of your interviews appropriately. To help you plan effectively for the residency matching process, we have created the following timetable to guide you through your third and fourth years.

April and May of Your Third Year

- Begin to inquire about "away" electives at other medical schools (optional).

- Start familiarizing yourself with the training program options in specialties and locations of interest utilizing the American Medical Association's updated online resource, the Fellowship and Residency Electronic Interactive Database Access System (alias AMA–FREIDA).
- Begin meeting with faculty advisors to discuss your thoughts on specialty selection and how you may be able to utilize your fourth year rotations to help make or reaffirm this decision.
- You might also tap into the experience of senior students to discuss your fourth year schedule and the upcoming application process.

June and July (Transitioning from Your Third Year to Fourth Year)

- Continue to familiarize yourself with the training program options in specialties and locations of interest utilizing the AMA–FREIDA system, and start identifying programs of interest by reading about them online.
- Continue to seek individual counseling from faculty attendings and residency advisors, in addition to current house staff who most recently went through the residency application and selection process.
- If possible, "test the waters" with electives in specialties of great interest to solidify your specialty selection.
- Begin requesting letters of recommendation from faculty members who you feel know you the best (you may also do this earlier in your third year while memories are fresh from clerkship attendings).
- Be sure to familiarize yourself with registration deadlines and application requirements for all matching programs, including the National Resident Matching Program (NRMP), and, if applicable, other independent matching programs (for example, at the time of publication, postgraduate training positions in Urology are filled through a separate matching program through the American Urological Association, and positions in Child Neu-

rology, Ophthalmology, and Plastic Surgery are filled through the San Francisco Resident and Fellow Matching Programs).
- Application photos should be taken.

August and September of Your Fourth Year

- Continue individual counseling with faculty advisors.
- Continue to familiarize yourself with programs online, and with the assistance of your advisors, establish a preliminary list of programs to which you will apply.
- Continue to be aware of early application deadlines.
- Continue to solicit letters of recommendation from faculty members.
- Begin preparing your personal statement once you feel comfortable that you have decided upon an area of specialization (do not be anxious if you are still uncertain).
- If you are applying through the San Francisco Matching Programs for positions in Child Neurology, Ophthalmology, and Plastic Surgery, the target dates for receipt of application materials by the Central Application Service are usually near late August.
- You may begin transmitting your Electronic Residency Application Services (ERAS) application materials at this time.

October and November of Your Fourth Year

- Continue individual counseling with faculty members and residency advisors.
- Ideally, your ERAS application should be transmitted to the ERAS Post Office by early October.
- Some programs will allow you to schedule interviews before receiving your MSPE, and others will wait to review your MSPE before extending invitations to interview.
- The interview season usually begins in early to mid-November and extends through late January.

- If you are applying for postgraduate year 2 (PGY-2) positions (whether through the NRMP or through one of the Independent Matching Programs) in addition to PGY-1 positions (through the NRMP), please try to schedule both sets of interviews on the same trip.
- MSPEs will be released on or after November 1 as mandated by the Association of American Medical Colleges.
- Applicants should be enrolled in the NRMP by the end of this time window (usually before December 1 of your fourth year of medical school).

December and January of Your Fourth Year

- Continue to seek advice from faculty members, residency advisors, and current residents.
- Continue the interview process.
- The ranking and matching processes for Child Neurology and Ophthalmology usually occur in January of your fourth year of medical school.

February of Your Fourth Year

- Continue to seek advice from faculty, house staff, and internship advisors as you finalize your rank lists.
- Interviewing in most cases will be winding down; however, this is a time when you might like to make second visits to programs of greatest interest (optional).
- Consider sending follow-up letters to programs (optional).
- Begin entering your NRMP rank list online, and be sure that you're aware of all deadlines.

March of Your Fourth Year

- Match Week usually occurs in the middle week of March.
- The Scramble Process usually begins mid-day Eastern Time on Tuesday of the middle week of March.

- Match results are usually released at 1:00 PM Eastern Time on Thursday of the middle week of March.

SUGGESTED READINGS

American Medical Association Fellowship and Residency Electronic Interactive Database Access System (AMA–FREIDA). Chicago, IL: American Medical Association. Updated annually. *http://www.ama-assn.org/ama/pub/category/2997.html*.

American Medical Association. *Graduate Medical Education Directory*, American Medical Association, published annually and may be ordered online at: *http://www.ama-assn.org/ama/pub/category/3991.html*.

American Medical Association Student Research Forums. *http://www.ama-assn.org/ama/pub/category/8247.html*.

Darrow V. The "audition" elective. In Langsley D. (Ed.): *How to Select Residents*. Evanston, IL: American Board of Medical Specialties Publishers, 1988:49–59.

Englander R, Carraccio C, Zalneraitis E, Sarkin R, and Morgenstern B. Guiding Medical Students Through the Match: Perspectives From Recent Graduates. *Pediatrics*, 2003:112;502–505.

Iserson KV. *Iserson's Getting into a Residency: A Guide for Medical Students*. 7th ed., Galen Press, Tucson, AZ, 2006.

Strolling Through the Match, hosted by the American Academy of Family Physicians News and Publication available at: *http://www.aafp.org/online/en/home/publications/otherpubs/strolling.html*.

3

The Matching Process

There are generally four different paths of residency application. This chapter outlines the particulars of each one, including the National Resident Matching Program (NRMP), the United States Armed Forces Match, Advanced Specialty Programs with their own matches, and programs that select their residents from a direct application process.

NATIONAL RESIDENT MATCHING PROGRAM

The vast majority of positions for graduate medical training will be filled through the NRMP. This program offers the applicant the opportunity to rank residency programs independently and confidentially in order of preference. Similarly, residency selection committees are given the opportunity to rank the candidates who have chosen to interview at their institutions. The final outcome is that each applicant is matched to the training program highest on the applicant's rank order list that has offered the applicant a position and has not filled its positions with applicants preferred by the program. Applicants must register to participate in the NRMP, and a complete directory of all participating programs is available online to all registered applicants. Additional information for both senior students enrolled in medical schools in the United States and independent applicants may be found on the NRMP web page at *http://www.nrmp.org*.

Applicants must meet requirements established by the Accreditation Council for Graduate Medical Education to enroll in the NRMP. Senior students enrolled in U.S. allopathic medical schools accredited by the Liaison Committee on Medical Education (LCME) are eligible for registration. Graduates of these schools, along with students and graduates of Canadian medical schools, students and graduates of schools accredited by the American Osteopathic Association, and students and graduates of international medical schools who hold an unrestricted license to practice medicine in a U.S. jurisdiction or who have fulfilled the requirements for certification by the Educational Commission for Foreign Medical Graduates (ECFMG) are also eligible to participate. You should consult the NRMP web page for a more detailed description of the rules and regulations of the NRMP.

CATEGORIES OF PROGRAMS WITHIN THE NATIONAL RESIDENT MATCHING PROGRAM

The NRMP offers several different categories of matching opportunities, as outlined below. These include categorical programs, transitional programs, preliminary track programs, and advanced specialty programs.

Categorical Programs

Categorical programs offer positions that begin in the first postgraduate year, with no requirement for previous postgraduate medical education. Most categorical programs are 3 to 5 years in duration and ultimately lead to eligibility for Board certification upon successful completion of the programs.

Transitional Programs

Transitional programs provide the resident with 1 year of preliminary training that encompasses multiple specialties. For example, this type of residency may include rotations in internal medicine, emergency medicine, general surgery, pediatrics, obstetrics and gynecology, and psychiatry during the first postgraduate year. Transitional year programs are designed to provide broad clinical experience for those medical school graduates who think that such experience will provide a strong foundation for subsequent graduate medical education (e.g., in anesthesiology or radiology). The Association for Hospital Medical Education supports the Council of Transitional Year Program Directors, and you may access their most up-to-date Directory of Transitional Year Programs at *http://www.ahme.org/publications/transitional.html*.

Preliminary Tracks in Internal Medicine, General Surgery, and Pediatrics

Like the transitional year programs, preliminary tracks in internal medicine, general surgery, and, in some cases, pediatrics provide the resident with 1 to 2 years of postgraduate training in each discipline. Residents applying for such tracks are not seeking Board eligibility in those specialties, but rather 1 to 2 years of training in clinical medicine that may serve as a prerequisite for subsequent postgraduate medical education in other disciplines (e.g., anesthesiology, radiology, and otolaryngology).

Advanced Specialty Programs

Advanced specialty programs begin in the second postgraduate year and require 1 year of preliminary track training in internal medicine, general surgery, or pediatrics or 1 year of transitional year training. Those programs usually commence the year following the match year. Applicants ranking such programs are provided the opportunity to link compatible PGY-1 residencies (transitional year programs or preliminary year programs in Medicine, Surgery, or Pediatrics) if a match results. Examples of programs that may require such preliminary training include orthopedic surgery, diagnostic radiology, anesthesiology, ophthalmology, dermatology, psychiatry, and emergency medicine. Some but not all institutions will offer candidates 1 to 2 years of preliminary or transitional track training if accepted into their advanced specialty programs. Applicants to advanced specialty programs may assign supplemental rank order lists of preliminary programs to each advanced program. Much of this information is detailed for you in the most recent edition of the *Graduate Medical Education Directory* published by the American Medical Association and summarized for you as well by the NRMP on the following web page: *http://www.nrmp.org/res_match/about_res/index.html*.

SPECIAL MATCHING OPPORTUNITIES WITHIN THE NATIONAL RESIDENT MATCHING PROGRAM

The NRMP offers several special matching opportunities to meet the personal or professional needs of some candidates. These include the following:

Shared-Schedule Positions

A very small subset of programs will allow two residents to share one full-time position by alternating the months when each house officer is on service. For example, a traditional 3-year primary care training program may take two residents a total of 6 years for both house officers to meet the requirements of Board eligibility. Programs offering such shared schedules are identified in the American Medical Association Fellowship and Residency Electronic Interactive Database Access (AMA–FREIDA) system, and these specific programs should be contacted directly for specific details. Applicants interested in shared-schedule residency positions must enroll individually in the NRMP and contact the NRMP for further instructions. For more information on shared-schedule positions, we refer you to *http://www.nrmp.org/res_match/special_part/us_seniors/shared_residency.html*.

Couples

The NRMP provides the opportunity for any two applicants to rank programs as a couple, and, ultimately, to match them with programs suited to their needs. Each partner applies as an individual, except that the two partners must agree on the parameters that fit their needs. Because of this constraint and to maximize the number of interviews offered to them, individuals who participate in the Match as a couple tend to increase the overall number of programs to which they apply. They may rank the same program several times to create different "pairs" of programs with their partner. Partners must be honest about their choices in two important respects. First, they must consider the competitiveness of each partner with respect to his or her choice of specialty and be realistic about their chances of matching in their chosen specialties. Second, if a match is not likely for one partner, partners must decide which one should go unmatched so that the partners can be assured of staying together. For more detailed information on the couple's rank order lists, including instructions on the ranking process and ramifications for supplemental rank order lists, we refer you to *http://www.nrmp.org/res_match/special_part/us_seniors/ couples.html*.

If possible, it is beneficial for partners to interview in the same city at the same time in order to share the experience of the hospitals and the city. Occasionally, only one partner will be invited to interview at a hospital where the specialties of both partners are represented. Because an interview is almost always necessary to match with a program, some students have shared these circumstances with the respective program directors in an effort to secure interviews for both parties.

Combined Training Programs

In recent years, there has been a very dramatic increase in the number of combined-specialty resident training opportunities. A complete listing of these programs may be found on the AMA–FREIDA system. At this time, such training options include the following:

- Combined Internal Medicine/Dermatology—These programs offer 5 years of combined training, acceptable to both the American Board of Internal Medicine and the American Board of Dermatology toward certification.

- Combined Internal Medicine/Emergency Medicine Programs—These programs offer 5 years of combined training, $2^1/2$ years in each specialty, acceptable to both the American Board of Internal Medicine and the American Board of Emergency Medicine toward certification.
- Combined Internal Medicine/Emergency Medicine/Critical Care Medicine—These programs offer 6 years of combined training, acceptable to both the American Board of Internal Medicine and the American Board of Emergency Medicine toward certification.
- Combined Internal Medicine/Family Medicine Programs— The American Board of Internal Medicine and the American Board of Family Practice offer dual certification for candidates who have satisfactorily completed 4 years of combined training in programs approved by both boards.
- Combined Internal Medicine/Medical Genetics Programs— These programs offer 5 years of combined training, acceptable to both the American Board of Pediatrics and the American Board of Medical Genetics toward certification.
- Combined Internal Medicine/Neurology—These programs offer 5 years of combined training acceptable to both the American Board of Internal Medicine and the American Board of Neurology.
- Combined Internal Medicine/Nuclear Medicine—These programs offer 4 years of combined training, acceptable to both the American Board of Internal Medicine and the American Board of Nuclear Medicine toward certification.
- Combined Internal Medicine/Pediatrics Programs—These programs offer 4 years of combined training, 2 years in each specialty, acceptable to both the American Board of Internal Medicine and the American Board of Pediatrics toward certification.
- Combined Internal Medicine/Physical Medicine and Rehabilitation—These programs offer 5 years of combined training, $2^1/2$ years in each specialty, acceptable to both the American Board of Internal Medicine and the Amer-

ican Board of Physical Medicine and Rehabilitation toward certification.

- Combined Internal Medicine/Preventive Medicine—These programs offer 4 years of combined training, acceptable to both the American Board of Internal Medicine and the American Board of Preventive Medicine toward certification.
- Combined Internal Medicine/Psychiatry Programs—These programs offer 5 years of combined training, acceptable to both the American Board of Internal Medicine and the American Board of Psychiatry and Neurology.
- Combined Neurology/Diagnostic Radiology/Neuroradiology—These programs offer 7 years of combined training, acceptable to both the American Board of Psychiatry and Neurology and the American Board of Radiology toward certification.
- Combined Pediatrics/Dermatology—These programs offer 5 years of combined training, acceptable to both the American Board of Pediatrics and the American Board of Dermatology toward certification.
- Combined Pediatrics/Emergency Medicine Programs— These programs offer 5 years of combined training, acceptable to both the American Board of Pediatrics and the American Board of Emergency Medicine toward certification.
- Combined Pediatrics/Medical Genetics Programs—These programs offer 5 years of combined training, acceptable to both the American Board of Pediatrics and the American Board of Medical Genetics toward certification.
- Combined Pediatrics/Physical Medicine and Rehabilitation Programs—These programs offer 5 years of combined training, acceptable to both the American Board of Pediatrics and the American Board of Physical Medicine and Rehabilitation toward certification.
- Combined Pediatrics/Psychiatry/Child Psychiatry Programs—These 5-year programs include 2 years of training in pediatrics, $1^1/_2$ years of adult psychiatry, and $1^1/_2$ years of child and adolescent psychiatry.

- Combined Psychiatry/Family Medicine—The American Board of Family Practice and the American Board of Psychiatry and Neurology offer dual certification in family practice and psychiatry. A combined residency in family practice and psychiatry must include at least 5 years of coherent training integral to residencies in the two disciplines.
- Combined Psychiatry/Neurology—The American Board of Psychiatry and Neurology has established guidelines for combined training in Psychiatry and Neurology. A combined residency must include PGY-1 training that is acceptable to neurology, plus a minimum of 5 years of combined residency training. The 5 years of residency training are usually taken at one approved institution, but may be taken at no more than two approved institutions.
- Combined Surgery/Plastic Surgery—These programs are integrated programs in which residents are matched directly into plastic surgery. Their 5 years of combined training may include some plastic surgery rotations during the first 3 years of their general surgery training.

For more information regarding any of the preceding training opportunities, you may contact the Specialty Board offices or may address your questions to the program directors at individual institutions.

THE UNITED STATES ARMED FORCES PROGRAMS

The Army, Navy, and Air Force have their own graduate medical education training programs that do not participate in the NRMP. Applicants to such training programs must be qualified for appointment as commissioned officers in the Armed Services. Positions may be filled by graduates of accredited schools of medicine and osteopathic medicine, or by U.S. citizens who are graduating from non-U.S. and non-Canadian medical schools, provided they are certified by the ECFMG. Most first-year graduate medical education positions in the Armed Services are filled by individuals with existing active duty service obligations. We recommend that applicants to the Armed Services program apply to the NRMP as well, as there may be fewer military residency positions available than the number of applicants vying for these positions. The Armed Services communicate directly with the NRMP so that if you obtain a military position you will be automatically withdrawn from the NRMP Match. For additional information, contact your local Armed Services recruitment officer.

ADVANCED SPECIALTY PROGRAMS WITH THEIR OWN MATCHING PROGRAMS

There are some specialties that have established their own matching programs for resident selection. Applicants who match through advanced specialty matches must not participate in the NRMP Match for positions beginning at the same time, but may participate in the NRMP Match for a preliminary year program. U.S. allopathic medical school senior students who obtain advanced positions through another matching program must participate in the NRMP to obtain their preliminary positions. Please also note that some specialties offer training positions through both the NRMP and through the independent matching process, and we recommend consulting with your medical school Dean of Student Affairs Office for an updated list of such programs.

There are two independent matching services that have different timetables for application than the NRMP, as follows below. Applicants applying to programs utilizing these other matching programs are urged to study their web pages and understand fully the requirements and deadlines of each program.

THE SAN FRANCISCO RESIDENT AND FELLOWSHIP MATCHING SERVICES

As early as 1977, the San Francisco Matching Program began coordinating the ranking process for a subset of programs not participating in the NRMP, and now thousands of graduating medical students are participating annually in this service. More specifically, at the time of publication, the San Francisco Matching Service coordinates the ranking processes for 3 residency and 18 fellowship training programs, including those in Child Neurology, Ophthalmology, and Plastic Surgery.

For more detailed information on the application, ranking, and matching processes for each of these specialties, we refer you to *http://www.sfmatch.org*. In some cases the application routes may be extremely complicated and merit careful review and discussion with your faculty advisors. For example, whereas some plastic surgery programs will make "integrated appointments" at the PGY-1 level through the NRMP (offering 3 years of surgery and 2 years of plastic surgery by a single appointment), other appointments are handled by the Plastic Surgery Matching Program through the San Francisco Matching Programs. Once again, please make sure you have a thorough understanding of your application and training options. For a summary of all application and ranking deadlines for programs participating in the San Francisco Matching Services, we refer you to *http://www.sfmatch.org/general/general_timetable.htm*.

Please note that programs participating in the San Francisco Matching Programs may utilize a Centralized Application Service (or CAS). The details of each application process may vary by specialty and are referenced at the above link.

THE RESIDENCY MATCHING PROGRAM FOR UROLOGY

The American Urologic Association coordinates the residency matching program for those applicants to postgraduate training in Urology. In most cases, applications may be processed through the Electronic Residency Application Service (see Chapter 5). For more details on the application, ranking, and matching processes for training in Urology, we refer you to *http://www.auanet.org/residents/resmatch.cfm#general*.

Note that some programs in Urology will also participate in the NRMP to match applicants for their general surgery training years. For more specifics, we encourage you to request information on this from each individual program.

NON-MATCH PROGRAMS

Although the minority, some graduate training programs do not participate in any matching program, but rather select their residents from a direct application process. As application procedures may vary from year to year, we suggest that you contact the program directors directly (as outlined in the AMA–FREIDA system) for specific details on their application process on an annual basis.

SUGGESTED READINGS

American Medical Association, Fellowship and Residency Electronic Interactive Database Access System (AMA–FREIDA), Chicago, American Medical Association, updated annually. *http://www.ama-assn.org/ama/pub/category/2997.html*.

Graduate Medical Education Directory, American Medical Association, published annually and may be ordered online at: *http://www.ama-assn.org/ama/pub/category/3991.html*.

Iserson KV. *Iserson's Getting into a Residency: A Guide for Medical Students*. 7th ed., Galen Press, Tucson, AZ, 2006.

Le T, Bhushan V, Amin C, Berk S, Collisson E. *First Aid for the Match* (First Aid Series). 4th ed., McGraw Hill, 2006.

NRMP Web Page: *http://www.nrmp.org*.

Residency Matching Program in Urology: *http://www.auanet.org/residents/resmatch.cfm#general*.

Roadmap to Residency: From Application to the Match and Beyond, American Association of Medical Colleges. May be ordered online at: *https://services.aamc.org/Publications/index.cfm?fuseaction=Product.displayForm&prd_id=183&cfid=1&cftoken=FD244488-A2E9-448F-A530B78D08C5D840*.

San Francisco Resident and Matching Programs: *http://www.sfmatch.org*.

Strolling Through the Match, hosted by the American Academy of Family Physicians. *http://aafp.org/online/en/home/publications/otherpubs/strolling.html*.

Selecting Programs
for Application

The first step in selecting programs for application is to review an up-to-date listing of all programs in your specialty of choice that are approved by the Accreditation Council of Graduate Medical Education. You should become very familiar with the American Medical Association Fellowship and Residency Electronic Interactive Database Access (AMA–FREIDA) system, easily accessible through the AMA's general home page (*http://www.ama-assn.org*) under Medical Science and Education. During the summer and fall of each year, program directors of all accredited specialty and subspecialty programs are asked to submit detailed data on their programs, including information on the size of each program, work schedules, call frequency, features of their didactic curriculum, maternity and paternity leave policies, salary, and vacation policies. This information is updated on an annual basis. Each program listing will also include the email address of the individual who will respond to your inquiries. Hard copies of the *Graduate Medical Education Directory*, also known as the "Green Book," may be ordered directly from the AMA at *http://www.ama-assn.org/ama/pub/category/3991.html*.

HOW MANY PROGRAMS?

Most students will read online about a larger number of programs than those to which they will ultimately apply. For example, although this will vary from specialty to specialty, for some primary care areas you might initially consider 20 or more programs. You might transmit your application to 15 of these, interview at 10 of these, and perhaps rank only eight or nine of these programs. Again, and very importantly, the above numbers will vary from specialty to specialty, and your faculty advisors should be helpful in guiding you to choose the appropriate types of programs and the number of programs to which you should apply based upon the competitiveness of each specialty and based upon your academic record.

SETTING YOUR PRIORITIES

Every applicant for residency training will have a different set of priorities and goals. In the process of selecting programs for application, we strongly suggest that you carefully consider each program's academic environment and size. Do not ignore the surrounding community or environment outside of the medical center in choosing programs. We urge you to read about a large variety of programs so that you can better appreciate the multitude of options available to you.

Academic Environment

There is a wide variety of medical centers in which you may elect to train, ranging from academic university centers, to university-affiliated or community-based programs, to county medical centers, to programs based at Health Maintenance Organizations, and to training programs at Veterans Administration facilities. If you are seriously considering a career in academic medicine, you should concentrate on university programs or other programs where the faculty maintains very active teaching and research commitments. You may want to be even more selective in seeking programs with particular strengths in a subspecialty of great interest to you (for example, adult cardiology), provided the basic residency curriculum emphasizes a strong clinical foundation upon which you may build your academic career (e.g., broad-based training in general internal medicine).

Size

Although some training programs will attempt to impress you with the large size of their residency program and the accompanying huge clinical load, others will emphasize the more personal nature and closer attention offered by their smaller departments. We are certain that you can receive strong training in either environment provided you are offered robust teaching with an appropriate clinical load. It may be useful for you to divide the total number of inpatient admissions by the number of house officers in each program to make a fair comparison of patient-to-resident ratios. Although some interns appreciate a very high patient load to build confidence, others prefer a somewhat smaller patient volume with additional time available for teaching, reading, and conferences. We suggest that you read about programs of all sizes and then select programs that offer the "happy medium" of the above benefits to best suit your personal style and interests.

Surrounding Community

Do not underestimate the importance of geographic location in selecting programs for application. If you are unhappy with the surrounding community for whatever reasons (e.g., size, crime rate, lack of cultural opportunities, distance from home, lack of employment opportunities for your spouse or significant other), then you will not be able to maximize your training experience to the extent that you would if you were personally more satisfied with the surroundings outside of the medical center. Remember that as a house officer in most specialties (especially during the first postgraduate year) you will have a limited amount of time to enjoy away from the hospital. You must, therefore, maximize your free time by selecting the environment that will best suit your personal needs and interests.

SEEKING ADVICE

There are four excellent sources of advice readily available to you as you select programs for internship application. These include the Department Chair of the specialty of interest at your home institution, selected members of the faculty of the same department, senior medical students who are preparing for their own graduation and who have recently interviewed and experienced the matching process, and house officers at your home institution who have chosen the same specialty and may be able to share their impressions from their own relatively recent application process.

The Department Chair is usually attuned to trends in the academic community and may offer a unique perspective on the strengths and weaknesses of individual programs. The Chair may also be informed about very recent or upcoming changes at institutions that you are considering. For example, current information on Department Chair changes, faculty recruitment or losses, financial stability of the medical center, and clinical and research strengths may contribute to your overall assessment. A counseling session with the Chair in the summer or early fall will not only help you to focus on appropriate programs that best suit your needs, but also provides the opportunity to discuss a chairman's letter of recommendation, which may be required by some programs.

You should also seek out a faculty advisor who has significant experience in guiding recent graduates through the residency selection process. Many departments will assign this responsibility to a member of the faculty who may serve as a counselor for all senior students interested in pursuing their particular area of postgraduate study. If this assigned person does not meet your specific needs, you should feel free to seek out a different advisor. Such advisors should be able to provide a list of the institutions where recent medical alumni are currently training. Do not be shy about calling these recent graduates with such candid questions as: "Would you choose the same program if given the opportunity to rank programs all over again?" and "How does your program compare with the training available at our medical school?"

Medical students in the class ahead of you are frequently more aware of the current status of training programs than are either of the two previously mentioned resources. These students have visited the individual programs most recently and should be able to provide their perspectives on the various house staffs, the "esprit de corps" encountered with each visit, the competitiveness of each program, and other factors that you may not even have considered. Just before graduation, you may want to organize a counseling session for all third-year students interested in a particular specialty with the senior student counterparts who have already matched with such programs and are preparing to leave for their internships.

House officers (especially first-year residents) at your home institution may also be able to share their perspectives on programs that are of interest to you. Furthermore, they may have friends who are currently training at these centers and may provide an insider's view into the training programs' strengths and weaknesses. We cannot overemphasize the importance of speaking with those who are currently enrolled within training programs.

After tapping into the above sources of advice and establishing your priorities with respect to academic strengths, size, location, and atmosphere, by late summer or early fall you should begin to narrow down your list of programs from the AMA–FREIDA computer system. If by August or September you are still uncertain about which specialty you would like to pursue after graduation, then we suggest that you read about programs in all areas that you are seriously considering. This way, when you do commit yourself to a particular specialty by the late fall or early winter, you will have a preliminary list of programs in mind and will not further delay the application process.

Once again, most senior students will read in detail about more programs than those to which they will actually apply. Given the constraints of time, distance, and finances, it is unusual for senior students to interview at more than 12 to 15 training programs (although there is wide variability based upon the competitiveness of particular specialties and personal circumstances, including the Couple's Match). You may certainly elect to apply to many more programs initially and can later narrow down your interview list to only those programs that you believe will best suit your needs and interests.

SUGGESTED READINGS

American Medical Association, Fellowship and Residency Electronic Interactive Database Access System (AMA–FREIDA), Chicago, American Medical Association, updated annually. *http://www.ama-assn.org/ama/pub/category/2997.html.*

Graduate Medical Education Directory, American Medical Association, published annually and may be ordered online at: *http://www.ama-assn.org/ama/pub/category/3991.html.*

Iserson KV. *Iserson's Getting into a Residency: A Guide for Medical Students.* 7th ed., Galen Press, Tucson, AZ, 2006.

Le T, Bhushan V, Amin C, Berk S, Collisson E. *First Aid for the Match* (First Aid Series). 4th ed., McGraw-Hill, 2006.

Roadmap to Residency: From Application to the Match and Beyond, American Association of Medical Colleges. May be ordered online at: *https://services.aamc.org/Publications/index.cfm?fuseaction=Product.displayForm&prd_id=183&cfid=1&cftoken=FD244488-A2E9-448F-A530B78D08C5D840.*

Strolling Through the Match, hosted by the American Academy of Family Physicians. *http://aafp.org/online/en/home/publications/otherpubs/strolling.html.*

The Application

In years past, medical students were faced with the arduous task of completing individual applications for each residency training program. Now, however, for most residency training programs students will use the Electronic Residency Application Service (ERAS) developed by the Association of American Medical Colleges to facilitate the internet transmission of residency application materials as detailed below. For the most up-to-date listing of which specialties and which individual programs are participating in ERAS, please refer to *https://services.aamc.org/eras/erasstats/par/*, or to the Applicant Support Section of *http://www.aamc.org/students/eras/*.

ELECTRONIC RESIDENCY APPLICATION SERVICE

The ERAS transmits residency, fellowship, and osteopathic applications, along with supportive credentials, directly to

Program Directors via the internet. More specifically, the transmitted materials include your application and personal statement, which you will prepare at home and transmit to programs via ERAS; your letters of recommendation, Medical Student Performance Evaluation (MSPE), medical school transcripts, and other supporting credentials that are submitted on your behalf to ERAS by your designated Dean's Office; and your Comprehensive Osteopathic Medical Licensing Examinations or United States Medical Licensing Examination transcripts, which may be transmitted directly to ERAS from the National Board of Osteopathic Medical Examiners or the National Board of Medical Examiners upon your request. The ERAS Post Office is essentially a bank of computers that transfers all of the above application materials to the programs of your choosing. By logging onto the Applicant Data Tracking System, an applicant may monitor the activity of his or her electronic application file.

In order to be able to complete application materials online, each student may obtain access to his or her individualized ERAS web site (known as the "My ERAS Web Site") by requesting an electronic token from the student's designated Dean's Office. With access to the "My ERAS Web Site," students may then complete their application and personal statement, and also select programs on this site to which they would like to apply. Ultimately, their application materials will be transmitted from the ERAS Post Office to these programs. ERAS, in turn, charges a fee to each student for this service, based upon the numbers of programs selected within each specialty.

Concurrently, each student's designated Dean's Office is using the "Dean's Office Workstation" to scan and submit supportive documentation to accompany the application and personal statement submitted by each student. Such documentation usually includes the applicant's transcript, letters of recommendation, photograph, and MSPE.

Program Directors also have software enabling them to download information transmitted to them by the ERAS Post Office (this was the information previously submitted by students via the "My ERAS Web Site" and by the designated Dean's Office via the "Dean's Office Workstation"). On a regular basis, each program can download newly transmitted application materials to make sure that each applicant's file is fully updated.

For more detailed and updated information on the ERAS, please refer to *http://www.aamc.org/students/eras/start.htm*, as well as the other links referenced below. What follows are some targeted suggestions on the individual components of your application.

Application Personal Statements

While some programs may ask you to answer very specific questions on supplemental application materials, most will only require you to submit a universal personal statement as part of your ERAS application materials. This is a great opportunity for you to share information about yourself and your interests. A wide variety of issues may be raised in your personal statement, including the following:

- Why you are selecting a particular specialty, or why you feel particularly well suited for the specialty to which you are applying.
- What you are looking for in a residency training program (i.e., what are your priorities for your postgraduate training experience).
- At this point in time, what long-range career plans are you considering after your residency training, and whether you are now leaning in a particular direction

(e.g., academic medicine, private practice, public health, or working for a Health Maintenance Organization).

- You may include an autobiographical sketch summarizing your undergraduate years, family, etc., especially if these things have had a strong impact on your specialty choice.
- If applicable, what are your research accomplishments, publications, and/or projects that may highlight your intellectual curiosity, and perhaps may have resulted in special recognition from the academic community?
- You may include extracurricular activities and passions (including community service projects that might highlight your humanistic qualities, hobbies, cultural interests, etc.).
- You may include unusual adventures, travel experiences, or outside interests.
- Any combination of the above.

You should not feel as though you need to discuss all of the items in the preceding list. Any combination may be appropriate, although at an absolute minimum, you should address why you have chosen to pursue your training in a particular specialty or subspecialty. Do not feel as though you must include a very detailed description of your upbringing or family history unless you would like to share with the reader how your earlier years may have contributed to your professional development and current career choice.

Please do not fill a page repeating all of the information that will be included on your curriculum vitae, which will be submitted along with your other application materials. The personal statement does, however, provide an opportunity for you to expand upon those particular items listed on your curriculum vitae that are worthy of highlighting.

We also want to caution you against making your personal statement another medical school application essay, thus telling the reader all of the factors that stimulated you to pursue a career in medicine.

It is also very important for you to communicate briefly some outside interests in your personal statement. In evaluating your credentials, a residency selection committee might appreciate knowing about your non-academic extra-curricular activities, including such things as family, sports, travel, foreign languages, film, theater, reading, music, and dancing. For example, if you have had an unusual hiking adventure in the Himalayan Mountains or have gone bungee-jumping over the Zambezi River, then share this information in your personal statement. A two to three sentence description of these outside interests usually placed at the end of your personal statement may serve as a great springboard for a relaxing conversation with an interviewer who may share similar interests (i.e., an "ice-breaker" to help you to feel more comfortable and at ease).

Your personal statement should be clear, concise, and articulate. This statement need not have a theme nor be particularly eccentric or flashy. Although we encourage creativity, we caution you that extremely unusual personal statements run the risk of being viewed negatively by some readers. Avoid non-professional comments such as "Ever since I began carving the Thanksgiving turkey at age 12, I knew that I wanted to be a surgeon" or "I knew I wanted to pursue a career in obstetrics at age 10 when I watched my pet beagle give birth to a litter of puppies."

We recommend that you try to condense your thoughts to no more than one typed page, as longer personal statements may not be read in their entirety by interviewers or by application screeners. For recommendations on formatting and font, please refer to *http://www.aamc.org/ students/eras/guideline/05.htm#ps*.

The final draft of your personal statement should be proofread carefully for typographical, grammatical, and spelling errors. All typing should be neatly and professionally prepared with appropriate margins and spacing. We encourage you to ask your faculty advisor to review your essay (some faculty members may wish to have a copy of your personal statement in addition to your curriculum vitae before composing a letter of recommendation). Remember, this is your opportunity to "shine" on paper. As an applicant, if you don't present yourself neatly and articulately when you have a lot of time to prepare your personal statement, what will your admission and progress notes be like when you are running around, busy on call? If you are uncomfortable with your writing skills, please be sure to have others review your personal statement before you send it.

Letters of Recommendation

All applicants for residency training will require a letter of recommendation from the Dean's Office (now known as the MSPE). Generally, your Dean of Student Affairs, or his or her designee, will complete this letter that summarizes your background, your performance in the basic sciences, your performance clinically (including comments from each of your core clerkships), and a bit about your extracurricular interests and/or activities. If you'd like to familiarize yourself with the format and content of the MSPE, please refer to *http://www.aamc.org/students/eras/resources/downloads/mspeguide.pdf*. Please note that there is a national policy that MPSEs are not mailed out until November 1 of each year.

In addition, many applications will require a letter from a Department Chair (or his or her designee) in addition to two or three other letters of recommendation. Unless you think that many different members of the faculty have significantly different perspectives on your performance, it is not wise to solicit more letters of recommendation than those requested by each program. Remember, a thicker application file does not necessarily make for a stronger file, so please don't go overboard soliciting extra letters. At the same time, you should not feel that all letters of recommendation must come solely from faculty members within the specialty to which you are applying. In addition to your MSPE and Chair's letter, a reasonable approach would be to solicit three additional letters of recommendation with at least one or two of these letters from members of the faculty within your specialty of interest. A letter from a faculty member in the Department of Internal Medicine is often helpful because Internal Medicine is universally considered to be a rigorous third-year rotation. It may also be to your advantage to solicit your letters from more senior members of the faculty who may be known by others within their specialties at the regional and national levels. The greatest priority in selecting faculty to write on your behalf, however, is to choose faculty members who know you best. Please do not ask someone to write for you if you did not share a strong working relationship, or if you feel that the person will not be able to assess your abilities accurately.

Once you have selected faculty members to submit letters on your behalf, you should schedule an appointment to meet with each of these people early in the application process (usually by September). It is polite and appropriate to ask each person if he or she knows your abilities well enough to submit a positive letter of recommendation on your behalf. If so, you should discuss your career goals and, at the same time, solicit advice about programs to which you should apply (see Chapter 4).

Each faculty member who agrees to write a letter of recommendation for you should receive an up-to-date curriculum vitae and a copy of your personal statement.

Most faculty members will also have access to your academic records in the Dean's Office should they require additional information on your performance on other services or in the basic sciences.

You must plan ahead in soliciting letters of recommendation with at least several weeks of advance notice to each faculty member before requesting that your letters be submitted to your designated Dean's Office (for subsequent submission to ERAS). Many programs will not even screen your application file, and therefore, not invite you for an interview, until your application is complete (including receipt of most letters of recommendation). Remember that faculty members may take vacation during the summer or early fall months and may be unavailable to you for solicitation of letters. To avoid some of these delays, you should solicit your references as early as possible at the start of your fourth year. Some students have even requested recommendations as early as their third year as they finish a clerkship with the faculty member in question (that is, provided they have performed well on the service and have had significant exposure to the attending involved).

The Curriculum Vitae

For the great majority of programs participating in the ERAS, the information from your curriculum vitae will be submitted in a template format provided by ERAS. You should, however, prepare a curriculum vitae for those faculty members that will be submitting letters of recommendation on your behalf.

There are many different styles and formats that you may use for preparing your curriculum vitae for this purpose. Regardless of the format selected, your resumé should provide for the reader a neat, concise summary of your academic and extracurricular activities, in addition to some basic biographical data. In most instances, your curriculum vitae should be condensed to one or two typewritten pages, without long, distracting text explanations of your employment, extracurricular activities, and research involvement. We have included a "sample format" (Figure 5.1) to assist you in the preparation of your resumé. Once again, you may choose among many different formats as long as your curriculum vitae is neat, well organized, and complete.

Some medical students will be elected to the Alpha Omega Alpha Honor Medical Society during the fall of their fourth year after ERAS applications have been transmitted and after curriculum vitaes have been distributed to faculty members writing on the student's behalf. If this is the case, you should update the individual faculty members, and ensure that all programs are also updated immediately on the change in status of your application. The latter is usually accomplished via ERAS by your designated Dean's Office.

Transcripts

Applications for residency training will require a copy of your medical school transcript, which will be transmitted by your designated Dean's Office. For significant changes in your transcript during the fall or winter months of your fourth year, you may request that updated versions of your transcript be transmitted to be sure that programs are aware of your most recent performance.

Application Photograph

The ERAS application will provide you with the opportunity to submit a recent photograph along with your other application materials. Although often optional, transmitting your photograph is a very helpful way to refresh the memories of interviewers and ranking committee members weeks to months after your actual interview date. Be sure to dress appropriately and professionally for this photograph. Casual photos on the beach, on camping trips, with pets, and in tee-shirts are not appropriate for this purpose. After receiving your Match results in the spring, many programs will request another photograph to prepare "photo rosters" for all incoming house staff.

Additional Tips for Your Application

Some lines of questioning on application materials may not apply to you specifically. For example, not every applicant has conducted research, yet the ERAS application will provide space for you to summarize your research activities (and also your publications). Do not worry about leaving these sections blank if you have no research experience and have not published.

Please also keep in mind that registering for ERAS is a separate process than registering for the various Match processes (whether through the National Resident Matching Program, through the Osteopathic Match, through the Military Match, through the San Francisco Matching Programs, or through the independent Urology Matching Program).

Please take advantage of the many resources that are available to you should you have any questions about the application process. In addition to experienced individuals within your Dean's Office, please tap into the multiple online and other references listed below.

Figure 5.1 Sample curriculum vitae.

JOHN DOE
CURRICULUM VITAE

<u>**Home Address & Telephone**</u>
123 Main Street
Apartment A
Hometown, USA 00000

<u>**Contact Information**</u>	<u>**Biographical Data**</u>
Home Phone:	Date of Birth:
Cell Phone:	Place of Birth:
Email:	Marital Status:

<u>Education</u>
2005–2009 —Medical School, City, and State
　　　　　 —MD anticipated in May, 2009
2001–2005 —Undergraduate Institution, City and State
　　　　　 —Degree earned, major (and Greek honors if applicable)

<u>**Honors and Awards**</u>
Date　　　 —Name of Honor and Award, followed by Name of School
Examples:
2008　　　 —Medical Alumni Scholarship, Name of Medical School
2005　　　 —Phi Beta Kappa, Name of College

<u>**Certification**</u>
United States Medical Licensing Examination, Step I
Month, Year—Three Digit score and Percentile
United States Medical Licensing Examination, Step II CK
Month, Year—Three Digit score and Percentile (or Pending)
United States Medical Licensing Examination, Step II CS
Month, Year—Passed (or Pending)

<u>**Research Experience**</u>
Date—Title of Investigation, Supervisor, location
Example:　2007—Investigation of (title of research project)
　　　　　 under _____ MD,
　　　　　 Dept. of _____, Name of Medical School

<u>**Publications**</u>
(Use standard reference format)

<u>**Extracurricular Activities and Employment**</u>
Date—One-line summary of each activity and/or job

<u>**Memberships**</u>
2005–2009—American Medical Student's Association

<u>**Outside Interests**</u> _____, _____, _____, _____.

SUGGESTED READINGS

Application materials for Urology Residency Programs: *http://www.auanet.org/match/urology/*.

ERAS Application Brochure: *http://www.aamc.org/students/eras/resources/downloads/applicantbrochure2008.pdf*.

ERAS Application Fees: *http://www.aamc.org/students/eras/feesbilling/start.htm*.

Important Application Deadlines for ERAS: *http://www.aamc.org/students/eras/timeline/start.htm*.

Iserson KV. *Iserson's Getting into a Residency: A Guide for Medical Students*. 7th ed., Galen Press, Tucson, AZ, 2006.

Le T, Bhushan V, Amin C, Berk S, Collisson E. *First Aid for the Match* (First Aid Series). 4th ed., McGraw Hill, 2006.

Roadmap to Residency: From Application to the Match and Beyond, American Association of Medical Colleges may be ordered online at: *https://services.aamc.org/Publications/index.cfm?fuseaction=Product.displayForm&prd_id=183&cfid=1&cftoken=FD244488-A2E9-448F-A530B78D08C5D840*.

MSPE: To familiarize yourself with the format and content, please refer to: *http://www.aamc.org/students/eras/resources/downloads/mspeguide.pdf*.

The San Francisco Matching Programs: *http://www.sfmatch.org/*.

Strolling Through the Match, hosted by the American Academy of Family Physicians: *http://aafp.org/online/en/home/publications/otherpubs/strolling.html*.

6

Interviewing

SCHEDULING TIPS FOR INTERVIEWS

Most fourth-year medical students schedule a 2- to 4-week block of time between November and late January for interviewing, depending on the number and distance of the programs to which they are applying. Early planning is essential as you begin the internship interviewing process. You will find that many programs will not even schedule appointments until all of your application materials are received (including all recommendations and your Medical Student Performance Evaluation). Therefore, if you are planning to interview in November, you may need to politely encourage faculty members to send their letters of recommendation to your designated Dean's Office for timely transmission. Depending on the competitiveness of the specialty and the individual programs involved, many residency selection committees will prescreen their applications and offer interviews on an invitation-only basis. Once invited, you will find some programs to be less flexible than others with the actual dates available for interviewing. Some institutions will offer interviews throughout the fall and winter on selected days of the week only (for example, every Tuesday and Thursday), whereas others will offer an even more limited selection of interview dates (e.g., 1 or 2 days per month from November through January or February). It will be a significant advantage for you to plan ahead in scheduling your interviews to meet the scheduling constraints, particularly of the programs for which you are most interested.

Alternative day interviews or special considerations requested on your behalf may be viewed negatively by the program and may be less than an ideal visit for you. Special requests require busy residents and faculty to schedule interviews on days that they are slated to be doing something else. Programs where particular days are established for interviewing generally include an orientation from the program director or chairman, special tours arranged by house officers, interviews by scheduled faculty, and possibly lunch or another less formal opportunity to see the program. On alternative interview days you will be fortunate if you see the facility and have a brief faculty interview. Avoid getting "closed out" of interviews because other candidates have filled all available interview positions for a given date. Remember that there are only a limited number of interviewers available on any given date at any given program.

We recommend that you systematically list all of the programs to which you have been invited for interviews along with the available days for interviewing at each center. Such scheduling should begin by October or November regardless of whether you are planning to complete your interviews in the late fall or winter. It is probably wise to schedule your first interviews at programs of lesser desirability, because you will certainly become more polished and more comfortable with interviewing with added experience. You should also try to schedule at least one full day at each program. If, after scheduling an interview appointment, you decide that you would like to decline the interview invitation, please call the program to cancel so that other students may be accommodated. Please do not be a "no show" without canceling, as this reflects very poorly on you and your school.

TIPS FOR TRAVEL ARRANGEMENTS

Travel expenses will accumulate rapidly if you choose to interview at many centers far from your home city. Students in need of funds for the interview process should check with the financial aid office of their medical schools to see if any assistance is available. In addition, we can recommend several ways to help you minimize the costs of lodging and travel.

Before leaving home, you should consult your medical school Alumni Directory for the names, addresses, and phone numbers of alumni residing in the cities where you will be visiting. Not only may such alumni provide an "insider's view" into the training programs or institutions that you will be visiting, but you may be offered overnight accommodations at their homes to help defray costs. Administrative personnel at training programs may also be able to recommend inexpensive overnight accommodations that will be convenient to the medical center. Some programs may have arranged discounted rates for applicants staying at nearby hotels and motels.

Punctuality is extremely important, and all travel arrangements should take into account unanticipated delays. If you are traveling long distances and will be required to arrive at the institution in the early morning, we suggest that you arrive the evening before your interview to get oriented and to assure that you arrive on time.

PREPARATION TIPS

We strongly recommend that you participate in practice interviews with a member of the faculty at your home institution. Not only may these rehearsals help lessen your anxieties, but you may also be confronted with several unanticipated questions for which you will appreciate the extra time to prepare clear, well-thought-out responses.

You should receive email, written, or telephone confirmation for all of your appointments before you embark on your interview trip. If you do not, we recommend that you contact the interview coordinators at each institution to avoid any miscommunication.

It should go without saying that you should arrive on time. Also, you will want to bring an adequate supply of interview outfits to present yourself in a neat and professional manner. Regardless of how you are accustomed to dressing at home, at work, or at school, you do not want to be remembered by your interviewers for what you were wearing. Do not show up with blue hair, sneakers, and tennis shorts, even if they have an alligator on them. Although we make light of this topic with these examples, accessories should be in good taste and should not include a lucky rabbit's foot on a chain or worry beads.

It's very important to arrive well prepared. If you're not traveling with a laptop computer, be sure to pack hard copies of all online information from each program before you leave home on your interview trip. It is essential for you to review this information carefully on the evening or morning just before your visit. You should approach each interview day with at least a basic understanding of the information presented in these materials to maximize your experience at each center. This approach will minimize the chances of asking questions that are already answered clearly on the program's web page and will provide you with the opportunity to clarify areas of uncertainty. Arriving with some basic understanding of the institution and training program will also help you appear more interested, well versed, and very organized. Please make sure your questions are pertinent and well focused.

THE IMPORTANCE OF THE INTERVIEW

The interview provides the applicant with very useful information about the "esprit de corps" of the house staff and the milieu of the institution. At the same time, the interview provides the faculty with a valuable glimpse of the applicant's personality. Please keep in mind that in addition to answering your questions about their programs, interviewers are seeking to assess your maturity, your commitment to hard work, and your compatibility with the personality of their particular program.

TIPS FOR THE INTERVIEW

A mild degree of nervousness is not unusual and will most often be discounted by your interviewer. Try to remain calm and at ease with yourself without putting on false airs. The great majority of interviews will not be high-pressured interrogations but will provide the opportunity for a pleasant and mutually rewarding exchange of information. Once again, interviewers may be trying to assess your maturity, articulateness, professionalism, enthusiasm, and outside interests, along with your level of interest in the program. It is imperative to have your thoughts on your professional goals and choice of specialty organized beforehand. On rare occasions, you may be asked a factual question or asked to present a clinical case for your interviewer (just in case, be prepared with a brief and interesting case history).

Be sure to ask intelligent questions about the training program, as a lack of inquiry may be falsely interpreted as disinterest. You may want to have several questions in mind even before you begin your interview. Some examples include:

1. What are the greatest strengths and weaknesses of this program? (This is a vastly overused question and often conveys to interviewers that you have given no thought to the characteristics of their particular institutions. However, if you communicate your understanding of the program, this question can be asked in the context of subspecialties covered or deficient, research opportunities, house staff morale, and teaching, to name a few.)
2. What paths have most of your recent graduates taken following completion of their training?
3. What are you looking for in a candidate and how might I fit into your program?
4. Do you feel that the volume of patients seen on both the inpatient and outpatient services provides an appropriate patient load for each house officer?
5. Is there a pyramid system for promotion in your program?
6. What are the major research interests within the department, or, which divisions within the department have been the most productive within the investigative arena?
7. From what medical schools have your current residents graduated?
8. Are your house officers encouraged and given funding to attend any continuing medical education courses or conferences during the academic year?

9. Can you describe the structure of your continuity clinics and the extent to which the residents are excused from their other responsibilities to attend?

10. How did your residents do on their Board certification examinations?

11. What major changes are anticipated in the department and/ or medical center and in what direction is the program headed?

12. What is the financial stability of the medical center, and how are changes in health care delivery affecting this medical center? (This has become increasingly important, and we feel that this question should be addressed at least once during each program visit.)

13. How would you assess the level of camaraderie and "esprit de corps" among the residents? (Ask this question of both the faculty and house staff.)

14. What is the relationship between private admitting physicians and the house officers, and do the residents have enough independence in the management of the private patients?

15. What elective opportunities are available to your house officers?

16. How would you describe the teaching program?

17. When alone with the house staff, be sure to ask them if they would choose this program if they had to make the selection all over again.

18. Ask the house staff if the faculty and administration are receptive to their suggestions, versus being more dictatorial.

19. Ask the house staff about their outside interests. Do they have time to enjoy themselves outside of work? (This is of critical importance in assessing lifestyle issues and your compatibility with the program and its people.)

20. Ask the house staff about the adequacy of the hospital's ancillary services, as this may affect your available time for reading and learning.

21. What changes in the program do you anticipate over the next 5 years?

22. Ask the program director what he or she would change if one thing could be different about the training program.

23. What is the mentorship and advising system like within the program? (What is the extent to which residents receive feedback in a timely fashion?)

To prepare for your interviews, we suggest that you ask the following questions of yourself before your first interview. Develop your best possible answers to these questions even if you are uncertain. You should realize that everybody expects you to be goal-oriented, but not wholly committed to these answers, and your philosophy should reflect an openness to change based upon your residency experiences. Questions asked by interviewers may include:

1. What questions do you have for us about this residency training program?
2. What are your interests outside of medicine?
3. What are your plans for after your residency training?
4. Why have you chosen this particular specialty?
5. What aspects of this particular training program are especially attractive to you? Or, are there any aspects that particularly concern you?
6. Please tell me more about your outside interests, or, what do you enjoy doing on your days off?
7. What books have you read recently?
8. How would you describe your major strengths? And your weaknesses?
9. In which direction do you see this specialty heading in the next 10 years, and how can you contribute to this field?
10. What would you do if you did not obtain a residency position for next year?
11. How do you feel about working with private physicians, and have you had any such experience?
12. Do you prefer any specific geographic location, and why?
13. If there were any blips in your academic performance (repeating a course examination or the Boards), be prepared to address questions related to this (and, if applica-

ble, be prepared to articulate any special circumstances or life events at the time).

14. Please tell me about yourself.

TURNOFFS

Several factors will assuredly turn off your interviewers from the start, including a sloppy personal appearance, poor manners, and lack of maturity. Make sure you arrive promptly for your interview; if you are unavoidably delayed, you should call ahead and provide a good explanation for your tardiness. Do not be argumentative with the administrative personnel or anyone else involved in the matching process. Other turnoffs include overaggressiveness, overbearing behavior, strong prejudices, narrow interests, and condemnation of other specialties. Do not look at your watch repetitively throughout the interview. Do not emphasize "connections" or influential individuals and be prepared to accept constructive criticism.

TIPS ON ASSESSING THE PROGRAM AND COMMUNITY

It will be in your best interest to spend as much time as possible at any given institution to assess the house staff and faculty, both formally and informally. Take advantage of opportunities to revisit the wards and clinics to discuss the program with the house staff even after your official interviewing has been completed. Assess the level of satisfaction of the current residents and their sense of camaraderie and support. Ask them candidly whether they would choose the same training program if given the opportunity to decide all over again. Be sure to get the name and email address of at least one house officer at every program whom you may contact at a later date with additional questions. After the formal interview activities, you might want to roam around the wards or clinics to meet and talk with as many of the residents as possible. No brochure really tells you what the house staff think of the program. Very importantly, just stand on the sidelines and take in the whole environment, observing interactions between all members of the health care team.

With the rapid changes in health care today, it's important for you to carefully assess the patient base and financial stability of each medical center involved in the program. This is absolutely critical.

It is equally important to assess the community surrounding the medical center. Make sure you leave with a good feel for the cost of living, areas in which the house staff currently reside, employment opportunities for your spouse or significant other, and cultural and recreational activities.

All of your impressions should be recorded soon after leaving each training program. We assure you that the details of each center will soon be forgotten or confused if not committed to paper in an organized fashion. List the important positives and negatives in order of priority, including your impressions of the house staff, faculty, "esprit de corps," curriculum, geographic location, physical plant, and benefits. Be sure to record any questions that might be answered with a follow-up telephone call, email message, or letter to the program director or chief resident. Alternatively, you might consider completion of the Residency Program Summary Sheet (Figure 6.1), which should be completed on the same day or night after leaving your interview.

Once you have finished the interview process, you may want to consider revisiting a program if you have enough time, finances, and energy. Remember that your initial impressions may be based on subjective and random circumstances, and you may interpret things differently on a repeat visit (e.g., was your tour guide irritable and somewhat unfriendly after an exhausting and difficult night on call?). Most programs would be delighted to have you visit them again in either an informal or formal fashion.

Thank you letters or email messages after your interviews are appropriate, but certainly not mandatory. You may want to take the opportunity to express your appreciation for the time given to you; and if you are still honestly excited about a training program, explain very briefly your continuing interest. Such forms of communication also provide opportunities to include updated information about yourself.

Figure 6.1 Residency Program Summary Sheet.

RESIDENCY PROGRAM SUMMARY SHEET

Program _____

Interview Date _____

Name(s) of Interviewer(s) _____

I. Current House Staff
—Size _____
—Esprit de Corps _____
—Happiness _____
—Other Comments _____
_____
_____

II. Workload
—Call Schedule _____
—Patient Volume _____
—Level of Independence _____
—Time to Read _____
—Time to Attend Conferences _____
—Other Comments _____

III. Faculty
—Availability of Attending Staff _____
—Availability of Subspecialty Coverage _____
—Preceptors in Clinic? On Wards? _____
—Percentage of Full-time Teaching Faculty _____

IV. Education
—Who does the teaching (H.S., Faculty, Fellows)? _____
—Teaching Conferences (Grand Rounds, Clinical Conferences,
House Staff Lectures) _____
—House Officer Curriculum Requirements _____
(Required rotations vs. selectives vs. electives) _____
—What have the graduates gone on to do? _____
(Fellowships, Practice, HMO, etc.) _____

V. Medical Center
—Type of hospital _____
(Community vs. University vs. HMO) _____
—Financial Stability _____
—Ancillary Services _____
(Including venipuncture, transport) _____
—Laboratory Services _____
—Patient Information _____
—Primary Care vs. Tertiary _____
—Social and Socioeconomic Backgrounds _____

VI. Compensation
   —Annual Salary_____
   —Vacation Leave _____
   —Educational Leave (conferences, etc.)_____
   —Maternity and Sick Leave _____
VII. Community
   —Strengths_____
   —Weaknesses_____
VIII. Overall Impressions
   _____
   _____
   _____
   _____
   _____
   _____
   _____

SUGGESTED READINGS

Iserson KV. *Iserson's Getting into a Residency: A Guide for Medical Students*. 7th ed., Galen Press, Tucson, AZ, 2006.

Le T, Bhushan V, Amin C, Berk S, Collisson E. *First Aid for the Match* (First Aid Series). 4th ed., McGraw Hill, 2006.

Roadmap to Residency: From Application to the Match and Beyond, American Association of Medical Colleges. May be ordered online at: *https://services.aamc.org/Publications/index.cfm?fuseaction=Product.displayForm&prd_id=183&cfid=1&cftoken=FD244488-A2E9-448F-A530B78D08C5D840*.

Strolling Through the Match, hosted by the American Academy of Family Physicians: *http://aafp.org/online/en/home/publications/otherpubs/strolling.html*.

Ranking

For the National Resident Matching Program, all applicants and residency training programs will enter their rank lists via the web by late February of each year. Although applicants will have a different set of priorities as they assess programs to establish their own rank lists, we suggest that your number one priority be a strong training experience in an environment where you can be happy and thrive. Be sure that you like the "personalities" of all programs that you are ranking. In comparing institutions, you might be torn by many factors, including the size of the programs, the academic reputations, how graduates fare on board certification exams, and what percentage of the graduates pursue careers in academic medicine versus private practice. All of these aspects will collectively create a "gestalt impression" as to whether you would like to train in a particular setting.

In establishing such priorities for yourself, do not underestimate the importance of personal happiness for you, and, if applicable, for your significant other or family. After an interview day, some programs will just feel right to you, and you may not be able to articulate the reasons for this attraction or sense of appeal. Do not ignore this feeling; in fact, consider it to be one of critical importance throughout the ranking process. When you respond to this "gut feeling," be sure to review the information tabulated on your Residency Program Summary Sheet (see Figure 6.1) to be certain that you understand the specifics of each program that you are considering. To allay uncertainties, you may want to revisit programs that you are considering ranking. If this is economically impossible or not feasible, consider a phone call to the residency program director, current chief resident, or a current house officer to address any lingering doubts, issues, or concerns, or just to be reminded of the many reasons why you so favored a particular program.

Over the years, we have certainly shared the anxieties of so many of our own advisees as they have sorted out the ranking process. While we appreciate that it is easier said than done, we'd like to urge you to maintain your perspective on the process, and hope that the following analogy will be helpful to you in doing so:

In some ways, the process of choosing a residency program is like choosing dessert. When making your choice for this next "course" in your education, try not to lose your perspective. For most students who are wrestling with how to sort out the order of their top couple of choices, it is important to remember that the choice is not between apple pie and arsenic. Instead, it is more likely that you are choosing between apple pie and an ice cream sundae. Aspects of one program may be sweeter to you than aspects of other programs, and classmates may or may not share the same tastes or impressions of each program. Once you feel comfortable that you can receive fine training at each of your top choices (keeping in mind that every program has different strengths as well as weaknesses, and that there is always room for improvement at every program), your decision becomes a visceral one. Remember to trust your heart on this one.

In Chapter 6 we emphasized the importance of assessing the details of each program. After having looked at the details of each "tree," take a step backward and "take in the whole forest." We can't emphasize enough how important it is for you to ask yourself over and over again the following questions about each program:

- How did I feel there?
- Do I think I could fit in?
- Would I like to be part of that group of people?

Think about Match Day and picture yourself viewing your Match results for the first time. Try to register this emotional response and your anticipated level of excitement and factor these in when you make up your final rank order list.

Here are some other general tips for you to consider before establishing your rank list. Ranking a program is a commitment to train at that program if a match results. If you have any doubts, do not rank the program. It is far better for you not to match than to match at a program or in a city about which you have very strong negative feelings. If you are pursuing a competitive field, your competitiveness needs to be discussed frankly with your advisors. In this case, it is wise to have other options on your rank list, including other less competitive specialties. If you already know what subspecialty you would like to pursue after your residency, consider training programs with academically strong divisions in this subspecialty to provide you with both good teaching in this area and effective references for your subsequent fellowship training. If you are undecided as to whether you would like to pursue a career in academic medicine, then lean toward more academic programs to maximize your options upon graduation. If you are certain that you are aiming for a career in private practice and are still somewhat undecided between two programs, then consider geographic location as an important factor to establish ties within the medical community there. Additionally, do not be shy about aiming high by including very competitive programs at the top of your rank list. It should not be important to you how far down your match list you go before matching. It is a greater priority to maximize your training opportunities and to allow the computer to match your preferences with those of the programs. At the same time, be sure not to overestimate yourself. Regardless of how comfortable you may be that you will match at your number one choice, it would be prudent to include additional programs on your list (but again, only if you feel as though you would enjoy training in these other programs). You will not be penalized for including additional listings.

Confidentiality of rank lists must be maintained by applicants and by residency program directors. Applicants and programs may volunteer information about how one plans to rank the other; however, it is inappropriate for applicants to solicit information on their rank position from the institutions to which they have applied. Similarly, residency program directors should not apply any pressure on applicants. All too frequently, students are shocked and disappointed on Match Day after having been told by program directors that they would be the program's number one choice. Both applicants and residency program directors have the right to change their rank lists before the final deadline for submission to the National Resident Matching Program.

Please note that for those programs participating in the Child Neurology, Ophthalmology, and Plastic Surgery matches (through the San Francisco Matching Program) or those participating in the Residency Matching Program for Urology (through the American Urologic Association), we encourage you to review their respective web pages for rules on the ranking processes of these programs (see Chapter 3).

SUGGESTED READINGS

Iserson KV. *Iserson's Getting into a Residency: A Guide for Medical Students*. 7th ed., Galen Press, Tucson, AZ, 2006.

Le T, Bhushan V, Amin C, Berk S, Collisson E. *First Aid for the Match* (First Aid Series). 4th ed., McGraw Hill, 2006.

Roadmap to Residency: From Application to the Match and Beyond, American Association of Medical Colleges. May be ordered online at: *https://services.aamc.org/Publications/index.cfm?fuseaction=Product.displayForm&prd_id=183&cfid=1&cftoken=FD244488-A2E9-448F-A530B78D08C5D840*.

Strolling Through the Match, hosted by the American Academy of Family Physicians: *http://aafp.org/online/en/home/publications/otherpubs/strolling.html*.

Match Week

Match Week for the National Resident Matching Program (NRMP) occurs each year in the middle of March, and it is the culmination of the long process of residency selection. At noon Eastern Time (ET) on the Monday of Match Week, all applicants learn if they matched to a program through the NRMP. Although applicants are not given the specifics of where they matched, they can log on to the NRMP web site using their Association of American Medical Colleges (AAMC) identification and password to learn if they matched with a categorical program, an advanced specialty program, and/or a preliminary track program. It is not until 1 PM ET on the Thursday of Match Week when the actual match results are posted to the NRMP web site. Those students who learn on Monday that they were unsuccessful in the Match begin the Scramble Process, during which time unmatched applicants apply to obtain positions in unfilled programs. At 12 noon ET on Tuesday of Match Week, the Dynamic List of Unfilled Positions is posted to the NRMP web site, and at this time students may begin the Scramble Process. Shortly after this week, hospitals will send letters of appointment to matched applicants.

Many institutions will plan a celebration in conjunction with Match Day activities. It is appropriate for you to bring your spouse or significant other to provide support and to share your excitement as you receive your Match results.

Each year, approximately 93% of U.S. allopathic seniors successfully match to a postgraduate year 1 position. Furthermore, the great majority of those students will match with one of their top three choices. For the most recent Match statistics and trends over the last 5 years, including Match statistics for U.S. Senior Students, for U.S. Physicians participating in the NRMP, for Osteopaths, for U.S. Foreign Graduates, and for Non-U.S. Foreign graduates, please refer to the online data on the NRMP web page at *http://www.nrmp.org/res_match/data_tables.html*.

The unmatched applicant faces significant emotional turmoil and should connect as soon as possible with faculty advisors and representatives of the Dean's Office for counseling and assistance with the Scramble Process. Such students will meet with their Deans of Student Affairs to discuss alternative options for training when the list of programs with unfilled positions is released on Tuesday of Match Week. The respective Department Chairs or Clerkship Directors may also be available to help solicit placement with their colleagues at institutions with these unfilled positions. Please note that there are very strict rules about when this Scramble Process begins. It is not acceptable for negotiations to begin any earlier. Many programs that go unfilled are excellent places to train, and thus, unmatched students can do extremely well. For comprehensive data on Match results from recent years, including the percentage of filled and unfilled programs and positions within each specialty, we refer you to the NRMP's web site at *www.nrmp.org*, which includes Results and Data for the Main Residency Match, as well as program results for the previous five years. Go to *http://www.nrmp.org/data/index.html* to obtain the information.

As a reminder, applicants and hospitals matched through the NRMP are contractually bound to one another. Programs are committed to offer an official appointment to each matched applicant who has met their prerequisites and institutional employment conditions, and applicants are committed to enter the positions into which they have been matched. Failure to fulfill this commitment is a Violation of the NRMP Agreement, which must be reported and investigated by the NRMP. For more information on this, we refer you to the NRMP Match Participation Agreement at *http://www.nrmp.org/res_match/policies/map_main.html*.

OTHER MATCHING PROGRAMS

The San Francisco Matching Programs and the Residency Matching Program for Urology through the American Urological Association release their Match results on a different timetable than the NRMP. Traditionally, the Match results for Child Neurology and Ophthalmology are released in January of each year, and the Match results for Plastic Surgery are released in May of each year. For more specific and updated information on the release of Match results through the San Francisco Resident and Fellowship Matching Services, we refer you to *http://www.sfmatch.org/general/general_timetable.htm*.

Results of the Resident Matching Program for Urology are usually released in late January, and for more specific and updated information we refer you to the American Urological Association Match Schedule at *http://www.auanet.org/residents/resmatch.cfm#schedule*.

Similarly, Match statistics are updated online annually for each of these other Matching Programs. These data are password protected through the San Francisco Match Residency and Fellowship Matching Service for the Child Neurology, Ophthalmology, and Plastic Surgery Matches. For annual Urology Match Statistics we refer you to *http://www.auanet.org/residents/resmatch.cfm#statistics*.

SUGGESTED READINGS

Iserson KV. *Iserson's Getting into a Residency: A Guide for Medical Students*. 7th ed., Galen Press, Tucson, AZ, 2006.

Le T, Bhushan V, Amin C, Berk S, Collisson E. *First Aid for the Match* (First Aid Series). 4th ed., McGraw Hill, 2006.

NRMP Results and Data, National Resident Matching Program, annual publication. May be ordered online at: *https://services.aamc.org/Publications/index.cfm?fuseaction=Catalog.displayForm&cfid=1&cftoken=6DDA5667-61A2-4DDD-B35F4EEC9F809F08*.

NRMP web page: *www.nrmp.org*.

Residency Matching Program in Urology: *http://www/auanet.org/residents/resmatch.cfm#general*.

Roadmap to Residency: From Application to the Match and Beyond, American Association of Medical Colleges. May be ordered online at: *https://services.aamc.org/Publications/index.cfm?fuseaction=Product.displayForm&prd_id=183&cfid=1&cftoken=FD244488-A2E9-448F-A530B78D08C5D840*.

San Francisco Resident and Matching Programs: *http://www.sfmatch.org*.

Strolling Through the Match, hosted by the American Academy of Family Physicians: *http://aafp.org/online/en/home/publications/otherpubs/strolling.html*.

Tips for the International Medical Graduate

INTRODUCTION TO EDUCATIONAL COMMISSION FOR FOREIGN MEDICAL GRADUATES CERTIFICATION

An International Medical Graduate (IMG) is defined by the Educational Commission for Foreign Medical Graduates (ECFMG) as a physician who graduated from a medical school located outside of the United States, Canada, and Puerto Rico, regardless of citizenship status. The purpose of ECFMG certification is to assess the readiness of IMGs to enter U.S. residency and fellowship programs that are accredited by the Accreditation Council for Graduate Medical Education (ACGME). In order to accomplish this, the ECFMG is responsible for evaluating the eligibility of international graduates to begin residency or fellowship training in programs accredited by the ACGME. The key take-home point here is that all graduates of foreign medical schools must hold a valid ECFMG Certificate to be eligible to participate in ACGME-accredited graduate medical education programs. Before applying for postgraduate training, it is therefore critical that you study the ECFMG web site (*http://www.ecfmg.org*) to understand clearly the most up-to-date requirements for certification, as well as all of the steps of the application process.

REQUIREMENTS FOR INTERNATIONAL MEDICAL GRADUATES TO APPLY FOR POSTGRADUATE TRAINING POSITIONS IN THE UNITED STATES

As an IMG, in order to enter an ACGME-accredited residency or fellowship program in the United States, you must be certified by the ECFMG before you can enter the program. In order to be eligible for ECFMG certification, you must graduate from a medical school listed in the International Medical Education Directory (IMED), and your medical education credentials must be primary source verified by the ECFMG. Furthermore, you must satisfy all of the examination requirements before completing the application process. More specifically regarding the directory, the Foundation for Advancement of International Medical Education and Research compiles the IMED, a free, web-based listing of medical schools abroad that are recognized by the appropriate government agency (usually the Ministry of Health) in the countries in which the schools are located. For more detailed information and for access to this database, please refer to *http://imed.ecfmg.org*.

In addition to the above, the requirements for ECFMG certification also include passing the following examinations:

1. The United States Medical Licensing Examination (USMLE) Step 1 Examination
2. The USMLE Step 2 Clinical Knowledge (CK) Examination
3. The USMLE Step 2 Clinical Skills (CS) Examination

Please note that applicants for ECFMG certification may take the USMLE Step 1 Examination, the USMLE Step 2 CK Examination, and the USMLE Step 2 CS Examination in any sequence, provided that all other eligibility requirements are met. For more details on all of the above, please study carefully the ECFMG Certification Fact Sheet that is available to you online at *http://ecfmg.org/cert/certfact.html* and in the ECFMG Information Booklet.

STAYING UPDATED ON ALL APPLICATION REQUIREMENTS AND THE STATUS OF YOUR APPLICATION MATERIALS

It is critical that all international students and graduates of international medical schools stay abreast of the updated requirements for certification by the ECFMG, as well as the status of their application materials for certification. Several web-based resources include the following:

ECFMG Information Booklet

The web site *http://ecfmg.org/2008ib/contents.html* is an annually updated and comprehensive overview of the entire certification and application process. Applicants are urged to read this most carefully, as it contains detailed information on application requirements and the logistics of scheduling all of the required testing in a timely manner (to meet all deadlines).

ECFMG-Electronic Residency Application Service News

There is a free email service designed to provide Electronic Residency Application Service (ERAS) applicants with important updated information as it becomes available. You may subscribe at *http://ecfmg.org/eras/erasnews.html*.

ECFMG Reporter

ECFMG Reporter is a free internet newsletter that provides international medical students with as much up-to-date information as possible in areas of likely interest. For example, issues may include updates on testing deadlines, Match statistics from the most recent academic year, profiles of medical education systems of selected countries, etc. You may subscribe at *http://ecfmg.org/ reporter/subscribe.html*.

Online Applicant Status and Information System (OASIS)

Online Applicant Status and Information System (OASIS) is a web-based service that allows you to check on the status of all of your certification requirements and facilitates your ability to update your contact information, etc., online. You may access this at *https://oasis2.ecfmg.org/*.

THE ELECTRONIC RESIDENCY APPLICATION SERVICE PROCESS FOR INTERNATIONAL MEDICAL GRADUATES

For IMGs, the ECFMG coordinates for you the ERAS application process (the majority of programs require applicants to submit their applications using ERAS). In other words, the ECFMG serves as the "Designated Dean's Office" for all IMGs. After receiving your payment of the required fees, the ECFMG will issue you a Token (a 14-digit alpha-numeric identification code) that will allow you to access the ERAS web site to complete your ERAS application online.

Although you will be completing your ERAS Common Application Form and Personal Statement online and transmitting these directly to ERAS, you will need to ensure that clear, sharp copies of all supporting documents are mailed directly to the ECFMG for subsequent transmission to ERAS on your behalf (using the ERAS Document Submission Form, which may be accessed at *http://www.ecfmg.org/eras/docform.pdf*). These include your Medical School Performance Evaluation, medical school transcript, letters of recommendation, and photograph. The ECFMG will scan these documents and transmit them on your behalf to the ERAS Post Office to be attached electronically to your application file.

After ERAS electronically mails out your completed application to the schools to which you are applying, it is then the responsibility of program directors to periodically retrieve all transmitted data from the ERAS Post Office.

As you begin the application process it is important for you to understand and anticipate all fees, including the following:

ECFMG Token Fee

The ECFMG token fee is a charge for the ECFMG to serve as your "Designated Dean's Office" (in other words, to scan your supporting documents and to transmit your ECFMG status report). For more information please refer to the ECFMG OASIS at *https://oasis2.ecfmg.org/*.

ERAS Processing Fee

ERAS charges a fee for serving as the postmaster for your application materials (with a sliding scale of fees according to the number of programs to which you're applying). For more information please refer to *http://www.aamc.org/students/eras/feesbilling/start.htm*.

USMLE Transcript Transmission Fee

There is a fee related to the transmission of USMLE transcripts from the ECFMG to ERAS. For more information please refer to *http://www.ecfmg.org/usmle/transcripts/index.html*.

National Resident Matching Program Registration and Ranking Fees

Please remember that enrollment in the National Resident Matching Program (NRMP) is a distinct process from enrollment in ERAS. For detailed information on all fees and specifics, please refer to *http://www.nrmp.org*.

It is also critically important that applicants are aware of all deadlines throughout the application process. Please remember that students and graduates of international medical schools must have passed all examinations necessary for ECFMG certification by the February deadline for submission of rank lists in order to remain in the NRMP Match system. The NRMP will communicate directly with the ECFMG to confirm that Match participants have passed the necessary examinations. Applicants who have not met the ECFMG requirements by the ranking deadline will be withdrawn automatically by the NRMP. It is therefore of critical importance that you plan carefully and understand your deadlines to ensure that you leave enough time for your scores to be reported to the NRMP.

Please review the information summarized on the ERAS application process in Chapter 5. There are some differences, though, in the application process for IMGs that merit highlighting:

ECFMG Status Report

In addition to the application requirements outlined for graduates of allopathic and osteopathic medicine, IMGs must also have an ECFMG Status Report transmitted to all programs (by the ECFMG).

California Application Status Letter

IMGs applying to programs in California will need to obtain a California Application Status Letter that should be forwarded to the ECFMG for transmission to ERAS, and ultimately to each residency program in California. More specifically, you may include the California Application Status Letter as one of the letters of recommendation that you would like to have forwarded to programs in California. Please keep in mind the time requirements of the Medical Board of California to review your credentials and to prepare this letter. For more detailed information on the California Application Status Letter, we refer you to *http://www.medbd.ca.gov*.

ECFMG Application Processing

The ECFMG processes your request for your USMLE transcript to be submitted to ERAS (versus U.S. allopathic students who make this request directly to the National Board of Medical Examiners).

ADDITIONAL TIPS FOR THE INTERNATIONAL MEDICAL GRADUATE

In addition to meeting the preceding general requirements for applying to residency training programs within the United States, we strongly recommend that IMGs contact the individual licensing board within each state to which they are applying for residency positions. Each state's licensing board may establish its own regulations concerning postgraduate training requirements and license eligibility, and these regulations are subject to change without notice. For a complete list of the names, addresses, and phone numbers of each state's licensing board, please refer to The Federation of State Medical Boards web page at *http://www.fsmb.org*.

Foreign nationals are responsible for fulfilling the requirements for obtaining the appropriate visas in order to participate in ACGME-accredited training programs. You may review information on the ECFMG Exchange Visitor Sponsorship Program (J-1 Visa) at *http://ecfmg.org/evsp/index.html*. As visa requirements and procedures may change, please check this site for updated information, as well as U.S. embassies and consulates of the U.S. Department of State (*http://usembassy.state.gov*), and the U.S. Department of Homeland Security (*http://www.dhs.gov*).

It should go without saying that all materials submitted should be neatly typed (see guidelines for the application process as outlined in Chapter 5). If English is not your native language, please be sure that your application materials, and most especially your personal statement, are reviewed by others before transmitting them to the ERAS.

We'd like to emphasize the importance to IMGs of obtaining constructive letters of recommendation from U.S. faculty references, which might be more easily interpreted by U.S. program directors than recommendation letters from sources abroad. In late 1989, the American Medical Association reminded all directors of residency training programs of their responsibility to evaluate all applicants carefully on the basis of their individual qualifications, in consideration of their knowledge, skill, and performance. The American Medical Association House of Delegates adopted a policy that explicitly states that it is inappropriate to measure the quality aspect solely on the basis of the country in which the medical education is received. With this in mind, it is extremely difficult for a residency program director to screen and interpret the credentials of all international graduates who are applying with such varied backgrounds. Most program directors will have little knowledge about the international graduate's level of competency upon completion of her or his undergraduate medical education, especially when considering that the training may be from one of a myriad of educational systems around the globe. Therefore, it becomes increasingly important for the IMG to submit references from U.S. faculty members who can speak to your abilities working in clinical settings that are quite similar to the environment in which you will be training in the United States.

On the curriculum vitae it may be helpful for IMGs to clarify their citizenship, and, if appropriate, their visa status.

SUGGESTED READINGS

2008 Information Booklet-ECFMG Certification, Philadelphia, Educational Commission for Foreign Medical Graduates Publishers, 2008: *http://www.ecfmg.org/2008ib/contents.html*.

Sammons JH. *Letter to Directors of Residency Programs*. American Medical Association, November 6, 1989.

Vora AA. *The Successful IMG—Obtaining a U.S. Residency*. Blackwell Publishing, Massachusetts, 2005.

Index

Note: Page numbers followed by *t* indicate tables; those followed by *f* indicate figures.